Strength Training 101

A Beginner's Guide To Gain Muscle and Lose Weight Easily

By: Kathy Cho

Introduction

I want to thank you and congratulate you for downloading the book, *"Strength Training 101"*.

This book contains proven steps and strategies on how to apply strength training strategies into your life even with limited time to spare towards it.

A beginner's guide is a little different than most books. It's meant to provide general rules in broad strokes to allow people to work it into their lives. This book is here to help new people explore strength training and start to explore new ideas for living a healthier and stronger life. I've included a nice glossary of possible terms that you may run into while interacting with other members of the strength training community either online or in person. It covers things like safety and the very basic things you'll need to start strength training and maintain the good habits successfully, leading you towards a path of lasting success with new healthy habits.

Thanks again for downloading this book, I hope you enjoy it!

The trademarks that are used are without any consent, and the publication of the trademark is without permission or backing by the trademark owner. All trademarks and brands within this book are for clarifying purposes only and are owned by the owners themselves, not affiliated with this document.

Table of Contents

What is Strength Training?

First, we almost have to start with the definitions that are going to be needed with the book. The thing about strength training is that it can mean a lot of things to a lot of different people. It can get a little hard to navigate the wild world of the internet to find the right words to explain what's going on, or to find classifications that tell you if something will actually work for you or not. We all know everyone is different, and some websites and books can be pretty vague on the subject. It's a sad truth, but one of them. And sometimes this book may seem to be a little bit vague, there simply isn't enough space to try to explain a way to solve every single issue you might run into. It simply isn't feasible for anyone to do this, it would take far to long, but with a variety of research, it's possible to get a good overview.

For the purpose of this book, I want to make it very clear that I'm not writing about bodybuilding. That's not what strength training really is anyway. It's about becoming stronger not building muscle mass. That may seem counter-intuitive, but it's the purpose of building yourself muscles that work more efficiently rather than make an impressive show. Not everyone wants to look like the Hulk, but a lot of us want to become more toned and have more strength in our day to day lives.

We've all seen body buildings, men and women that are stacked beyond belief. Something that seems impossible to reach. With this being the thought that most people think of it's easy to see how strength training can be intimidating. Not many people want to develop the bulk of bodybuilders, and understandably it's what a lot of people think about when its mentioned. It certainly was my first impression of the matter. When someone first talked to me about it, I was picturing the bulky bodybuilders that I watched on television all of those times. Normal strength training isn't quite like that, it's actually much less dramatic and filled with less powdered protein powder.

The thing with stuff like this is that it can be hard to find the right words to discuss it. Every day it's a struggle to describe what you're talking about to someone who doesn't know or to find someone who knows the right words to the things that you're describing. It's normal. Every new activity that we take part in has some kind of specialized jargon. You have to crack the jargon wall to really be able to get into it. A lot of people that are experienced don't even think about the jargon anymore, it's just ingrained in their habits and speech patterns. It stops people from getting into new things, the fear of not understanding what people are talking about. It's why I've included some of the beginner jargon that may help you get started.

These are natural challenges in trying to approach a new lifestyle, especially a healthier one. It's like learning a new language and stepping out of your comfort zone all at the same time, but there are ways to deal with the intimidating nature of beginning the process.

A big one is keeping in mind that you can strength train without going for bodybuilding, instead encouraging your muscles to work more efficiently. That's the goal of most people these days. A lot of us want to learn how to get stronger, sometimes it's just to pick up our kids as they start to get older. Sometimes it's for our health. Sometimes it for silly reasons like just wanting to look good on a date.

The truth is, that the reason that keeps you moving this direction doesn't matter so much as it matters to keep moving forward and keep fighting for that something better. For whatever reason you're really doing it, it becomes a habit that helps keep you healthy and stronger and that's worth keeping up. Just keep moving in a positive direction. You're bound to have a few hang-ups and problems as you go on, but don't let that stop you. Tomorrow is another day, and it may be hard, but if you make yourself move after a hiccup it only makes you stronger and stronger as time goes by.

So take a moment to congratulate yourself on a good decision and start to leaf through different techniques that I'm presenting here while you do more work to become a better version of yourself. A lot of places will tell you the first step in this process is to pick a reason that will resonate with you. It's easy to say that you want to be healthier, but it's more tangible to say that you want to fit into that pair of jeans you wore ten years ago or that you want to look nice in a wedding dress. These are the kinds of changes that stick with people, making a difference in the actual process. Having a tangible goal will help build the good habits that actually make a difference in your life. So, even if it's selfish, do it for a reason that will help you stick with it. For example, I started strength training to look better when I went to a high school reunion. A friend of mine did it because she wanted to stick it to her ex-husband. And yet another friend did it so he could pick up his kids more. There are thousands of reasons, but the important thing is to pick one that works for you and will work for you for the weeks or months it takes to develop the good habits that you need to keep going even after you get your goal.

Strength training can be a lot of fun too. A unique experience every time with a lot of different options out there to help everyone succeed at what they need to do. So, work with yourself to help yourself succeed. No one can make the perfect plan for you without knowing you, so unless you want to pay a small fortune for someone to put a plan together for you, it's vital to think about the goals you have in mind, put together a plan and then pick the right exercise to help you accomplish your goals.

Jargon! Ah!

You'll need some more definitions of course. It's hard to know what kind of help you might need without knowing the words.

Some of them will be used later in this text, but others won't. I added them anyway so that you can have them if you need them at other times. Not all books will have this kind of

information and if you're communicating with the community it may be hard to find the terms that you need. Keep in mind that each activity will have its own jargon, so each word may have a specific meaning in relation to the activity that it

doesn't have day to day. This causes a lot of people to get confused when they deal with a new activity. I know that I had this problem, so I figured I would offer this little glossary of jargon to start with. It should help when explanations get more complex later in your successful strength training.

Whatever the goals are, it's important to know exactly what

you're getting into, and part of that is learning the right jargon for the job.

Strength Training: The act of exercising in a controlled manner to promote the strengthening of existing muscle mass and tone down on excess fat on the body. This is not

bodybuilding and isn't to get stacked, but rather to tone and built tone musculature.

Rep: A rep is shortened for repetition. It's a completed motion through a single exercise. For example, a full push-up is a completed rep, starting at the upper position and down to the ground and back up. Usually, reps are counted out loud.

Set: A set is the number of reps of a specific exercise you do. Generally, it's grouped by rests. For example, if you do five pushups then rest, that's one set. If you take five pushups, rest, then do five more and rest again, that's two sets. And so on and so forth. The number of reps in a set varies due to your skill or ability to do them.

Rest: The pause you take between sets. Generally, these rests aren't very long. More often then not, the rests between sets are less than thirty seconds as not to fully drop down to resting heart rate, but sometimes it may be necessary to take longer rests.

Burn: The burning sensation that sometimes comes with intense exercise. It is actually from the build-up of lactic acid in the muscles. It's often described as 'feeling the burn'. Burn is a natural part of the process, so try not to let it frighten you. It isn't advised to let the burn get to extreme levels, but a little bit should be just fine.

Weight: The amount of resistance you add to a rep. For example, a thirty-pound dumbbell or a thirty-pound resistance band would both be called a thirty-pound weight. This is a way to describe the kind of progress your making in your strength training and can be a really good way to keep track of it all.

Intensity: The basic question of how much. How fast or how much stress you're putting on yourself. There are high intensity and low-intensity routines. High intensity may be with high weight or quick movements.

Volume: Another way to ask how much, but looking at the total number of sets and reps you can do during the entire exercise routine. In general, it's looking at the macro as compared to the intensity asking about the micro.

Frequency: How often you work on specific work out routine. It's the butt of a few jokes about not skipping leg day. If you work on your legs once per week, that's the frequency that you work on your legs.

Spotter: The person that watches and makes sure that you don't hurt yourself. Basically, spotters are only used when you're lifting heavier weights, as a way to make sure that you don't drop it on yourself and end up seriously injuring yourself. Most strength trainers don't require a spotter until they're using the equipment that can cause something to fall on the user if they're used wrong.

Positive Phase: To put it simply this is why you lift the weight, think of it going in a more positive direction. I like to call it the pick-up phase and think of it as the parts of the rep where I am actively working against gravity.

Negative Phase: This is when you lower the weight, controlling the descent with muscle control. I like to call this the put-down phase and think of it as the time's when I'm only controlling how gravity causes the object to descend.

Muscle Group: A group of muscles that work together to affect the same joint of the body. No one muscle controls the movement of a single joint, but rather the range of motion requires us to have different muscles that push or pull at certain times.

Stretching: The act of stretching a muscle or muscle group to its full extension. This aids in loosing up the muscle group before you start working with it. There are stretches that stretch every major muscle group.

Flexibility: A specific joint's range of motion, specifically measured as compared to the range of motion of the same joint at past times. As your training increases, you may find that your flexibility increases as well.

Exercise Routine: The specific number and intensity of certain motions required to maintain and/or improve upon physical health.

Circuit Training: Moving quickly from one exercise to another with very little rest between each set. A lot of this is moving from one set of each movement to a new movement almost immediately.

Cardiovascular: The heart and veins that pump blood and keep it working hard. Basically, the Cardiovascular System is the heart and blood circulatory system.

Peak Heartrate: The maximum heart rate that you want to reach over the course of an exercise routine. There is usually a ramp-up period, then a period of time you stay at the peak heart rate and then a cool down period where you slow down the exercising to allow your heart rate to slowly move back to the normal you stay at while resting. This may be repeated several times.

Bulking: This is the goal to reach higher levels of muscle mass. It's the sort of things that bodybuilders do to gain large muscular frames.

Cutting: Also called getting cut is the goal to get a more defined muscle mass.

Free Weights: The dumbbells or barbells that many people use to lift with. Basically, these weights are the weights that one would use that aren't attached to a machine. These are used primarily for bulking.

Machine Weights: Weights that are used as part of the resistance of a machine. Often these machines will mimic things that free weights can do with adjustable resistance, and occasionally they do things that would be difficult on free weights. These are the primary method for cutting.

Body Weight Exercises: These are exercises that use your body weight to your advantage. They have the added bonus of not requiring any equipment to do, thus they can be done anywhere that you have sufficient space. The premise that you use your own body weight to do the work of regular weight. A prime example is a push-up.

Pick and Choose

One of the most important parts of strength training is to identify exactly what you're going for and which parts of the body will be the major focus. This will allow you to research the right steps to take from the start so that you aren't wasting a lot of time and energy doing exercises that don't work for you.

This is the time when the difference between bulking and cutting comes into full sight. It's important to know which one you're aiming for from the get-go. For the purpose of this book, I'll be looking mostly at cutting, bulking is a much less popular form of strength training even if it is more widely viewed in the media.

It's important to know some specific goals when it comes to your body. Do you want to flatten your stomach or tone up your butt? A lot of people want to do both but to different degrees. This is where it becomes important to take stock of what level of importance each of your separate body goals is.

I usually help by making a list. Something like this:

1. Lose Weight

2. Strengthen Core

3. Flatten Stomach

4. Tone Legs

Then I rearrange them into the order that means the most to me. This usually takes some time and introspection on the matter, and sometimes it's just a matter of taking a list of pros and cons. Sometimes it's more work towards figuring out what's the most important.

The list will start to take a new order after you list the reasons why you want to accomplish these goals.

1. Flatten stomach.

2. Lose Weight.

3. Tone Legs and Buttocks.

4. Strengthen Core.

This list represents the major goal of looking better, perhaps for summer coming up or some other option for it. It's hard to tell what's most important to one person or another, so it's important that they find goals that work with them. Setting these goals help a lot with figuring out where to start.

Once you have the goals it's time to do some research in order to find what exercises and training will help you accomplish the goals. This is going to take some time, it always does, but I hope that you have some idea of how to start on that research.

The above example states that losing weight is most important so bulking shouldn't be the goal here. Bulking will cause you to gain weight due to increased muscle mass. While it will cut down the fat, most people aren't looking for giant muscles.

What you'll have to go for is cutting. It should fit beautifully into all of those goals, actually. Cutting will tone and strengthen existing muscle mass while the movements will help cut down excess fat. While it's not a fast form of weight loss, any sort of exercise should help with weight loss goals and it should help cut down pant sizes due to muscle weighing more than fat and looking more trim.

You may be able to mix some of the goals together, to work on one goal while you work on another at the same time. Losing weight may be a part of the exercises for the other goals, for example, it's very broad and can be done any number of different ways. So maybe we should look at the way the goal is written and make it a bit clearer. Maybe instead of focusing on losing weight, we want to focus instead on losing that excess fat that we're carrying around. That's fine. It's easy enough to work with, just keep it in mind when choosing the right circuits to do. This is important to keep in mind, so we start to adjust our goals once again. That means it's time to go back to the list we made, and maybe even add some more goals to specify better what we need to do.

1. Overarching Goal: Lose Excess Fat

    a. Flatten Stomach

    b. Tone Legs

    c. Tone Buttocks

    d. Strengthen Core

Our list has changed again, but that's fine. Now it looks like it all meshes together. While meeting the other goals you can be working towards the other goals at the same time, and that's great. Puts it all into something generally reachable. Any activity that increases more than one of the goals is something that should be worked towards and you can tailor the exercises of the secondary goals in order to make it all lead towards the primary goal. This is where it takes thought and careful planning.

The plan I presented here is very simplistic, and in no way should it be used in place of any one's personal goals. Very few people are going to start it with the same goals that I had in the beginning.

But let's say something changes and we decide that maybe we would like to bulk in certain areas.

These are a lot of things that can be kept in mind. But once you figure out exactly what you're trying to accomplish it gets to be time to work on finding the way to do it. You've got your plan set up now, so it's time to actually get started on losing the weight.

Start at Home!

Gym membership is so expensive. It should never cost as much as it does to use sweaty equipment that you never know the last time that it was used. It just feels wrong and icky, and adding to it is the fact that you're paying a lot of money to effectively have access to equipment. I wouldn't suggest starting at a gym myself, or even to start by buying a lot of expensive equipment. There are a lot of the exercises that you can do right from home.

You'll want to start directly with stretching. While there are a thousand different websites you can go to in order to check out stretches that you can do, there are some basics that are pretty easy.

With any stretching, it's important to slowly draw a muscle into full extension. Basically, stretching the muscle group. Every muscle group is going to have a different way to stretch, the problem being that you have muscles going in all different directions over your body, so it takes some effort to stretch all of them.

This also gets your body primed to exercise without hurting itself, which is definitely a good thing, so make sure to do those toe touches and leg stretches. Roll those shoulders.

I'll go through a few of my favorite stretches. One of my big ones is the Runner's stretch. This works for multiple muscle groups and also works on balance. You start off with a gentle lunging motion, one foot in front of the other in a wide stance and then bend the front knee. From this position, with your feet still in the same position from the lunge, you straighten the bent front leg, stretching out the muscles of the leg. You keep your hands on your front foot when you do this and it also stretches a This works really well, but make sure you switch front legs to get both of them the same way. This stretches out a lot of the muscles in the body at one time, so it's a decent time saver as well, just be sure to always pay attention to what your body is telling you. You don't want to strain or sprain anything.

Whenever you exercise at home, especially if you're alone it's important to pay attention to any kind of pain you feel. It may take some time to learn what's a natural level of discomfort from your actions, but don't be too shy to get started either.

The home is a great place to start. There are plenty of resources online to show you the proper form. Make sure to take a moment to check the sources, however, because it can be a little overwhelming when you're shown several different ways to do something.

As far as strength training, resistance bands are a great way to start toning and losing weight as well as running and climbing up and down stairs. None of this is expensive to start and could do a world of good. A lot of people have started doing simple things that are inexpensive to start. And the thing about it is, that if you can develop the discipline amid all of the distractions at home, being able to work out in a gym should be pretty easy for you.

Some people can't start at home, but if you can master the steps in your home environment, not spending the extra money you can make the whole process less expensive on you in the long run. Gym memberships and personal trainers are expensive. YouTube and Resistance bands are not. So its easier than ever to learn things as you go along, and work your way up to needing the kind of equipment that a gym can provide. The great thing about strength training is that most of the equipment for it is fairly small and inexpensive. This means great things unless you're at a more advanced level.

Plus, when you see your strength training not costing you a small fortune it can help you feel the effects even if you don't have the kind of money that hiring a professional takes. Let's face it, personal trainers can add up to exorbitant levels quickly. It's just the nature of the business.

I once actually watched a really neat documentary on strength training that used household items. Things like cans and bottles from the kitchen as free weights and stretchy belts for resistance bands. In no way is any of this stuff perfect, but for a beginner, it's a good idea not to waste a lot of extra money at the situation.

Anyway, that's just me. I like to add little money saving tips to things like these. Money is often such a huge factor for people trying to improve themselves, but if these tricks don't work for you, try to find the way that works best for you. Some people find that having someplace specific that they go to work out helps a lot, either a small home gym or a small place that they can go work out at. Others enjoy the support that a larger gym allows. The big important thing is that nothing is going to be the same for everyone. Each person has to take their own conditions and life circumstances into account.

There are a thousand other great ideas to do this starting in your home environment. It's my personal opinion that forming good habits in the places that you spend most of your time helps the habits stick with you. And this I feel is something that helps you maintain good habits, even if it makes it harder to start the process.

It takes willpower, all good changes in life do. The important thing is to develop good habits that last as long as you need them to. It's so easy to give up, so be sure to pick the way that will help you succeed the best. Everyone is very different in this regard, so it can be hard to do it to start.

Safety, Boring but Vital.

There is no way for me to stress this enough. Before you start anything like this, it is vital for you to speak to a doctor. It may seem like such a silly thing, but a doctor is going to be able to give you advice and maybe help you learn ways to work around the natural limitations of your body.

It's impossible to judge from a piece of paper or a simple internet search the kinds of things that you should be able to do from the start to prevent from hurting yourself. Again. Everyone is so very different.

This is especially important if you have some kind of preexisting condition before starting it. It's easy to make the kinds of mistakes that lead to injuries when trying to train your body to do something new like this. And mistakes do happen.

This is why it's important to go to a doctor and be honest with them. If your knee gives you occasional problems, this is definitely the time to bring it up. Let him do the testing and any checking he or she needs to do.

My own doctor insisted that I have x-rays done of one of my knees because I had a severe injury that required surgery. This is why it was so important. He was able to help me pick out a proper brace to wear while I worked out with it. I wanted to make sure that a chapter got into this book because it's so vital. Most texts on the subject mention it as a side note or it's in the small text at the bottom of any advertisement of a diet or exercise routine, but it's so much more important than anyone really makes it out to be.

It shouldn't be a side note. As with anything else, your health is important and it can't be stressed enough how much it means to do things that may lead to lasting injuries. Lasting injuries make lives so much more difficult.

Often times this will just lead to some braces or specific exercises to avoid. But for some people, it makes a huge difference. A friend of mine when to a doctor to get checked out for an exercise routine and was told that there was no way that she could start on anything so advanced. She had a skeletal condition that wouldn't allow her to do it safely.

The doctor suggested that she start with some sort of low-stress exercise until she was able to strengthen her joints. It started with a water aerobics class a couple times a week then gradually increased as she was able to handle more and more. It took months for her to work her body up to the kind of condition it would take to actually do strength training.

Still, she stuck with it, and can now keep up with most of the rest of our work out the group in various kinds of training. It just took her more time to get there. Because I've seen the kind of help that a doctor can offer someone that prevents the kind of horror stories that you can read about all over the internet. And those stories are all over the internet. They simply do not ever go away. You could go to any person and they could tell you about someone who made a serious mistake while working with exercise equipment.

On that note. If you are using exercise equipment it's so important to know how to use it properly. This may be when you actually go seek out a professional. Most gyms have people that you can ask specific questions like that too and there are always instruction manuals available out there for you to use, either with the equipment or available online. Be sure to look up anything that you may need. Your continuing ability to improve may rely on it.

Again. There are horror stories after horror stories about these kinds of accidents. Some of the worst involve some sort of falling equipment. This is a definite danger in home gyms and a partial danger in gyms who normally make sure that equipment is installed and set up properly.

The fall damage is easy to see because it's so shocking compared to normal injuries, but it's really the minor injuries that happen during a workout that add up to alarming levels. It's so easy to make mistakes that lead to someone getting hurt. This is why when using any sort of heavy equipment, it's important to use a spotter. Spotters can make the difference between success and failure in many instances too, watching form as well as immediately in range to help if something drops. This is one of the advantages that big gyms have over worked out at home. There are people there that can lend support and advice if you're using some piece of machinery right.

If you are doing the work at home, make sure to do plenty of research before getting started on any new exercise. Research form and take the time to learn to make the motions right so that you don't pull a muscle or strain something. Let's cover some of the basic exercises that you may do while I explain the ways to keep yourself safe when doing them.

On a bicep curl, you have a small weight in your hand. You sit on the edge of a bench and rest your elbow on your knee, careful to keep your back straight as you lean over. Keeping your arm straight, it's important to lift very carefully to make sure that you don't pull a muscle with the movement. Avoid jerky motions, and try to make a smooth arc using your elbow as a pivot. Make sure to keep the elbow solid, so that it does not move, but rather the rest of the arm moves around it. This will prevent many possible injuries.

Then there's the Goblet squat. You do this by holding a barbell out in front you. It's held like you would a cup or goblet, hence the name of the exercise. You hold it upright, by one end between your hands. Continue holding this dumbbell at arm's length, as if you're offering it to someone else standing with your feet shoulder width apart. Keeping your back straight, lower your butt until you are in a seated position without a seat under you. Hold there are long as you can comfortably before slowly rising back up. Again, make sure that you do this in a smooth motion, moving slowly to make a graceful arc.

Push-ups aren't as simple as they look from the outside either, but it's an old staple of strength training that focuses on the muscles of the upper body. Starting on your knees, place your hands directly under your shoulders to brace yourself. It's important for your support that you have your hands placed properly, shoulder-width apart and forming a right angle to the floor. Slowly straighten your knees so your weight is distributed on your feet and hands. From this position, keep your body straight, not sticking your butt in the air. This may require a spotter to help you find the right form. Slowly bend your elbows, once again, keep the movement smooth as you lower your weight towards the ground, your chest should very nearly touch the ground while doing this. Then slowly raise yourself back up. Once you're back in the starting position you've completed the rep.

The squat is another very basic exercise that many people start with. You simply start in a standing position with your feet shoulder width apart. Make sure to keep your back straight through the entire motion. You can do this with weights or without them, depending on your needs at the time. As you do the squat, bring your hands up to shoulder level, keeping your arms and back straight as you move into a position meant to mimic sitting in a chair. Then slowly raise back up to a standing position. Once you've completed the motion, you've completed a rep.

Another great exercise is a Lunge. The lunge is similar to the squat and works the lower body. Stand with your feet shoulder width apart, but you'll need to place one foot in front of the other, as if you're taking a single step, but paused before you bring the behind foot up. Doing this, take a moment to make sure that you are steady and in a smooth moment bend the front knee, keeping the back leg straight so you balance on the front leg using the ball of the back leg to steady yourself.

Smooth motions are important. Jerking around can cause injuries because you aren't in full control of the motions that you're making. If you cannot do an exercise without making jerking motions, it might be time to try a simpler version, something that's a lot easier for you to master, trying less weight or something to work yourself up to what you're trying to do.

Conclusion

Thank you again for downloading this book!

I hope this book was able to help you to start the process of strength training and lead yourself into a better life. There are a lot of little tricks that can help you work on your muscle tone and build a stronger body.

The next step is to follow the steps outlined in this book, and get started.

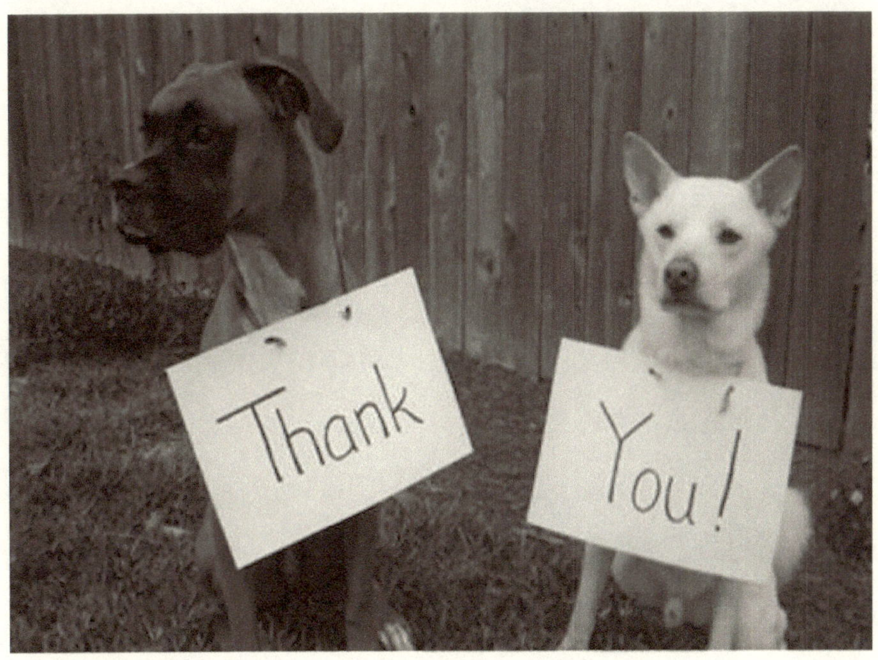

Finally, if you enjoyed this book, then I'd like to ask you for a favor, would you be kind enough to leave a review for this book on Amazon? It'd be greatly appreciated!

Thank you and good luck!